HIIT Your Way to Fit

HIIT Your Way to Fit

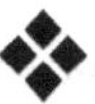

LaKeisha Jeanne Cole, Ph.D.

To order additional copies of this book, contact:
Xlibris
1-888-795-4274
www.Xlibris.com
Orders@Xlibris.com
810004

CONTENTS

This read is dedicated to my husband of twenty years (September), William Cole III, who has inspired me through the years to find my place in this world and understand that God has a greater plan and purpose for me to go well beyond what I would have for myself. I appreciate the experiences that taught me what I needed to be all I can be and move in the direction of positivity and success.

To our beautiful sons, William Cole IV and Khalil Cole who motivate me, you inspire me to write words of wisdom that will go on. My hope is that what I've learned from my failures in life will allow you to be successful, and my successes will be the foundation for you to achieve so much more. I always want the best for you. Thank you and I love you!

To all those individuals who have set health and wellness goals that they've never reached, I want you to know that you can do it! You must believe in yourself, discover what is hindering you from getting the results you desire and start making the change right now. Work hard and never give up on you and your dream health and fitness goals—it's achievable!

INTRODUCTION

In life, you have a responsibility to take care of yourself. In the beginning, you expect your parents to take care of you and ensure you get the best start in life to be healthy. When you're in grade school, you're introduced to sports or other physical activities that can support health. Sometimes you're interested, and other times you may not. Nevertheless, you must do something to ensure your physical well-being. As you grow older, it becomes significantly important for you to do what you can to maintain and sustain good health and well-being.

There is so much information in the world today about the importance of health and fitness. It can become overwhelming to the point that you may do nothing at all. What about the doctor's visits that stress the importance of eating right and getting exercise? There's that family history of disease—high blood pressure, high cholesterol, overweight and obesity, diabetes, and the list goes on. Oh, and don't forget those infomercials that get you excited about that exercise equipment designed to get you in shape and feel great, right?

Now there are new, more intense ways to train your body to get in better shape, such as high-intensity interval training, known as HIIT. Does it really work? How will it work for you? What role does it play in helping you reach your fitness and overall health goals? Should you even consider taking on another task? Will it be more *added to your plate* that appears exciting and new in the beginning but fails you when it comes down to maintaining the consistency necessary once it becomes a part of your daily routine?

Wow, so many questions to consider! Now, you have all these concerns on your mind about your health. And there are likely a few more. You probably have a busy schedule, too—no time for working out. If you do have the time, you probably don't feel like it—especially, if you have a job, children, spouse, and your personal *me* time.

But it's all necessary to stay fit, right? You must do it to be healthy, right? Oh my, don't you dare begin to overthink it— now, you're feeling stress—and that causes health problems, too, right?

Well, you must do something because your health and well-being cannot take a back seat in your life. No matter how you feel about it, you must take care of yourself. You are way too valuable in this world to neglect your health. And you deserve to feel good, be strong, and have the look you desire.

In this book, you will learn about what HIIT is and how it relates to your fitness goals. Also, you will learn the steps you need to take to enjoy a healthy life. You will have the opportunity to look at yourself and determine what role you play in living a healthy life. This book will offer you the guidance to understanding different lifestyle and health behaviors to consider for the results you've been searching for, in a quick, easy-to-read format. You will be provided with the motivation, inspiration, and encouragement to work at your own pace. Most importantly, you will be challenged to be consistent to ensure that you get results that will transform your life and how you feel about health and wellness. So let's get fit!

CHAPTER 1

Believe in Yourself!

In my book, *From Failure to Success: Faith Changes the Outcome*, I discussed the importance of having faith—believing in something greater than you which has the ability to get things done—anything you desire! Well, when it comes to your health, wellness, fitness, and overall well-being, you must use faith to believe that you can get the results you're expecting and beyond.

You must start with *you*! You must look yourself in the mirror and be truthful about what you believe is possible for you. What do you believe you can do concerning your health and fitness goals? Are you doubtful about being healthy and in the best shape of your life right now? Do you believe you deserve to be physically fit and have a life full of vitality and longevity? You must ask yourself these questions to discover what you believe you can achieve.

There is a lot of work to do, but you must first know what you believe to be possible for you before you begin. Being healthy takes work and time. You have a journey from where you are right now—physically, mentally, and spiritually. To be consistent with the necessary routines, life's changes, and unexpected things that may come your way to hinder your success, your belief will have the power to push you through when the tough gets going—and it definitely gets going!

What does your belief have to do with HIIT? Well, you must believe that you can do anything. Mentally, you must go there in your mind to know that you can do something new, different, and even a bit out of your comfort zone. You must convince yourself that you can and will benefit from this style of training. It's necessary to know that you deserve to do something that can take you to another level—a new level. Being physically fit requires strength on various levels. HIIT is all about taking your workouts to the next level, possibly one you've never attempted or succeeded before. Nevertheless, this is a new day, and you're serious about your goals and achieving your health and wellness dreams—and physical fitness is a part of that—and HIIT is definitely a part of that! Always remember that there is nothing that you cannot be, do, or have in your life. So believe and you will achieve!

Believe in Yourself: Positive Affirmations

I believe in the *power* within me. I believe in myself.

All things (according to the plan and purpose for my life) are possible for me to achieve.

I AM capable, willing, and able to do what I must do to get the best results possible for myself.

I shall achieve my health and fitness goals.

I AM getting in the best shape of my life, right now!

I deserve to be physically fit and have a life full of vitality and longevity.

There is a lot of work to do, but I AM ready for the challenge.

I AM willing to commit to the time it takes for my success.

I AM physically, mentally, and spiritually stronger than ever.

I AM prepared to succeed in my health and wellness goals.

HIIT is perfect for me. I can do it. I will be successful. I AM successful at HIIT!

I benefit from HIIT.

Today is a new day, and all that matters is NOW!

Remember, it is necessary to convince yourself that you can do anything. You cannot doubt yourself in any manner. It is okay to acknowledge your human thoughts about something new and particularly your health and wellness HIIT challenge. Nevertheless, you are preparing to be successful, and changing your thoughts is a significant part of the process. Before you begin, you must understand that it starts with your mind—what you are thinking and what you believe to be possible for you. If this seems strange to you—speaking the positive affirmations about yourself—do not allow that to discourage you from doing it. As you begin to speak the words, you need to know that you are putting those positive words of confession into the universe. You are stating your desire. As you continue to do this daily, you will become transformed in your mind. No matter what it has been before, you are taking control by speaking what you want and what it is now. You are taking specific action that must yield results. It may not seem like it at this time, but you will notice a difference in your attitude and how you feel as you continue.

It is the same practice necessary to form a habit. The more time you spend speaking positive affirmations over your life, the more you feel comfortable with it—remember to keep your mind focused in positivity mode because this is something important that you are doing for yourself. Do not allow that part of you that may be thinking, "This is silly!" or "This isn't going to change anything!" etc., to control you and keep your mind focused on the negativity which can hinder your progress. The beginning of every journey begins with a process that has a start and continues until the end—change must take place during the process of any transformation. Just know that you are making great progress!

CHAPTER 2

Consistency Is Key

Consistency is your ability to keep doing the same thing every day. You must be prepared to do the same thing each day, every week, and every month of this year. Then, you should be prepared to continue from there. No exercise program and nutritional support regimen will yield its best results if you are not prepared to *repeat* the cycle. You must be prepared to make this practice form a habit. Once you break through the inconsistent pattern in your mind and body, you will notice that your spirit has been guiding you along the pathway of success for your best results.

First, you want to have consistency in your state of mind each day. Every day when you rise, put healthy thoughts in your mind that you are on a mission to take your physical, mental, and spiritual body to another level—one of the highest levels you've ever achieved! Awaken with gratefulness that you are blessed to enjoy another day. Be thankful that you have found a resource that will help you reach your goals in health and wellness. Do not compare this health and wellness goal to any other you've had in the past. This is a completely new time in your life. Acknowledge and respect that you have never seen or lived this moment or day before. See this as a new opportunity every day. Do not fail to overlook your position in life on earth to make a difference—for you and others. In this moment, take time to physically look at your body and be thankful that it can perform now to undergo the process of transformation that is to come. All of this is vitally important! In order to be consistent in your mindful practice of appreciation, you must understand that you are making the steps. You are *doing* what it takes to physically see improvement in your life.

Second, you want to have consistency in your physical activity each day. Each day, you will be prepared to carry out some form of exercise routine to keep your body strong for the process. Yes, the process! This type of HIIT training requires taking your body to another level and requires physical adjustment. You will be engaging in different exercises that push your physical body in one area, and without rest—or very little—you will be moving to a completely different exercise that will work a different area. Your entire body will be actively involved in simple and complex movements at a fast pace, while at a slower pace over time. Nevertheless, it will be constant! You must be prepared to move, move, and move some more. Then, you will be held accountable to continue this routine daily, each day of each month (some of those days will include walking, only, to allow your body to recuperate), within a year—and this is just to break into a steady lifestyle habit that your body will appreciate. After that, you will mentally and physically be accustomed to this kind of training, and you can continue as you desire on your own terms over your lifetime. As with any program, once you reach your desired goal, you will move to a maintenance routine that will keep your body strong and conditioned for what it has already been trained to do.

Third, you must allow your spirit to lead you each day. This very important spiritual time is necessary because that part of you that does not want to take you to the next level will be riding your back, some days, trying to get you to quit! Each day, you must get in a quiet place and just allow your inner self to take over. Direct your focus on the good in life. Be in a position of willingness—to be guided. The power within you is the only thing that will get you guaranteed results. It will guide you through each day with the necessary preparation to fulfill the day's tasks. You may find that you have the mental and physical strength to be consistent with your consistency practice goals. You may also discover that you are ready or excited to push your body to the limit, whereas in the past you were not. Your spirit always wants the best for you. When you allow it to lead you throughout your day, there is nothing that you will not be able to do. There will be no challenge that you cannot overcome on any level. Make the time for no excuses to allow your spirit to guide you through this journey to your best results.

In conclusion, you must be prepared for the process of the journey. You will continue to have your daily routine outside of your workout regimen. If you're a spouse, you will continue to have your spousal duties. If you are a parent, you will continue to have your parental duties and responsibilities. Your job will have its place in your life as well. Each of these roles will require your daily time and have its own mental and physical stressors; nevertheless, you must ensure that your health and well-being is no less important. Remember, if you do not prioritize your health and wellness to ensure you will be up to the tasks of your other obligations, you may hinder your ability to be your best in other areas of your life that you believe matter most.

Consistency Is Key: Positive Affirmations

I AM consistent in my daily spiritual, physical, and mental routines.

I AM positively focused on improving mentally for my physical training program.

I will be successful in my effort to be consistent each day.

I will surround myself with positive people who support my physical training goals.

I AM consistent in my attitude to keep moving forward each day.

I AM consistent in my daily practices that will form positive lifestyle habits.

I will be prosperous in my family as I achieve my consistency fitness goals.

I AM willing to carry out my daily duties and responsibilities and improve my health.

I AM prepared for the journey ahead of me, and I will be successful.

CHAPTER 3

Focus Adjustment

Focus is something that you must be willing to possess before tackling the HIIT challenge. It is a challenge because you will be required to push yourself hard, in a way that you've never pushed before. It is necessary to be aware of distractions—in many different forms—that may try to take your attention away from your goals. You must practice focusing on your health and wellness goals, your daily practice routines for the mind, body, and spirit, and be prepared to keep moving forward if you find yourself distracted. In this chapter, you will discover what you focus your attention on and how to maintain fitness concentration in different atmospheres.

As you prepare to be challenged physically with high intensity, you must check your mental state for distractions. You have a life and there are many things that you must do daily. So find out what is on your mind, tackle it, and get ready to focus. Consider every important thing that you must do that will require your attention before you get ready to start training. Make sure you take care of every person that needs your time prior to beginning your workout. Inform those important in your life about what you are doing so they can offer their support—mainly for the respect of your time to train. You will not require much time, so prioritize what needs your attention from those things that can wait until your session is complete.

You must be prepared to guide your focus from the power within. As you arise each day, consider how you will begin your day on a mental level. Start by opening the door of your mind to determine what you are thinking about. There were probably thoughts running through your mind as you slept through the night—some peaceful dreams, hopefully, but maybe there were other thoughts that could have been stressful.

Well, it's important to know that you have control, first thing in the morning. You should gather yourself by taking a deep breath. Gain control over your thoughts and make the choice to think positively. You decide what you will give your attention to; it does not decide for you. Consider the fact that you are alive right now. You have been awakened for a special purpose today. Treat your focus control over your thoughts by using the domino effect. Whatever you are giving attention or focus through your thoughts will be written like a tablet on the imaginary domino of your mind. Choose your focus because what is written on that domino will soon fall forward on the rest of the dominos that determine your entire day. For example, you may focus your attention on how beautiful your day will be by saying, "Today is a beautiful day for me! Everything is working well for me. Good favor is flowing in my direction as I move throughout the day. What a wonderful day this is for me!" You may choose to write this message down in your notepad or in a text message to yourself. During conversation, use these phrases when speaking about your day and its activities.

What about the distractive thoughts that may come to try to disturb you? You must always keep in mind that you are in charge and you have the power to control your focus. Every thought that disagrees with you—refuse it! Allow that thought to pass and tell yourself what you will focus on. Then, whatever you are doing at that moment, continue doing it. For example, when you are working at your desk or doing something productive on your job and you notice someone is talking loudly and gossiping about the latest news—keep working! If you recognize that you have begun listening in, give yourself credit for being aware that your focus has shifted then get right back to what you know you should be doing—maintaining the focus of the domino effect. Another example, when you are engaging in your physical fitness routine and someone is watching or decides to start a conversation with you, keep your eyes on the equipment that you are using, which will help you to resist distraction of eye contact with anyone or anything other than it. Politely let the other person know that you have very little time, and you must get your workout completed. There are many different distractions, but just keep in mind that you must maintain focus. Every time you notice a distraction, keep regaining focus repeatedly. Do not allow the distraction to cause you to feel as if "this focus thing" isn't working out. Keep moving forward as many times as necessary because this is a practice that is forming a habit. It's okay; you're not alone. It happens!

Focus Adjustment: Positive Affirmations

I AM prepared for this day.

I AM focusing my attention on the things I desire.

I AM good at directing my focus.

I AM aware that I am in control of my thoughts.

I decide the direction of my focus and follow through with my thoughts.

I AM not easily distracted by negativity.

As I move through my day, I shall accomplish my tasks to completion.

I AM on the right focused path for my life.

I give my attention to things that I appreciate.

My attention is focused on my self-worth.

I AM aware that good thoughts will guide my focus to action.

These positive affirmations are examples of words that you can use to motivate yourself to take control of your focus. You may choose to use the positive affirmations that feel good to you. This is an important practice for your focus. You will be able to see how your mind wanders, or not, during this activity. If it does, this will be the focus practice that this chapter discussed. Remind yourself that you are practicing forming a healthy habit and keep going. Distractions may come, but that does not have to discourage you. It is a normal process of the mind, and you have the power to control it. If you continue to make the choice to follow through, you will soon become the master at moving forward through distractions. That is what focus is about—making the shift to turn the attention back to where you want it.

CHAPTER 4

Ready, Set, HIIT

Okay, now it's time! You've had a great head start. You have received a fantastic introduction to the mindset that is required to embark on this HIIT challenge. It might have seemed like a bit too much, but you'll soon see that motivation and inspiration is required for what is to come. As you begin this exercise routine and the complementary lifestyle practices that support its provision to yield the absolute best results, you'll understand why this book's first few chapters were necessary. You will need to refer to them daily to continue to serve as the encouragement to keep moving forward when it has broken through.

HIIT Defined

You need to know how HIIT is defined. What is it, and what does it mean? HIIT is an abbreviation for high-intensity interval training. This type of training can be considered a cardiovascular exercise support approach that consists of periods of intense anaerobic exercise (high energy demand *without oxygen* supply efficient enough for the activity and must use glucose as energy from the muscles) with very short periods of allowing the body to recover before moving to the next exercise. When exercising, your body requires energy to support physical fitness training to get your body to perform, burn unhealthy and undesirable fat, and decrease overall body-fat percentage, as well as build that beautiful lean muscle that will get you stronger than ever—all necessary to live life enjoyably to support daily activities and those other things needed to get things done—for yourself or just for having fun! Depending upon the duration of the exercise or how long the exercise is performed and the intensity or how hard you push the body through the exercise, this energy used to support the routine will aid the body in burning more fat during and after your workout is complete. Your body will receive this energy from the food that you have consumed, which provides calories or energy to support your physical activity demand. Just remember, your food provides the energy to support your ability to get through the workout—each exercise within the routine program for that day. You will be guided to better understand the importance of nutrition and the role it plays in exercise and fitness support in the next chapter.

Below is an example of one week's exercise routine centered around the HIIT concept and exercise plan. Your choice in use of dumbbell or other weights or not, as well as the specific weight in pounds depends upon your level of training readiness. Each exercise can be changed based on fit by design for your strength level. You may choose to increase or decrease the number of repetitions of each exercise and the sets performed according to your fitness level. Choose any five of the seven days of the week. A sample would look something like this:

Monday

Full-body circuit training for three to five rounds (completion of all exercises before rest of 45–60 seconds, then repeat cycle again for total of three to five times indicating one round)

20 kettlebell swings with 20 lb. dumbbells

10 burpees with or without ankle weights (2.5 lb. or more)

10 kettlebell squats with two 20 lb. bells (one in each hand equal to 40 lb.)

Isolation crunch holds with leg extensions (in

and out), holding hands at the sides of the ears with or without ankle weights (2.5 lb. or more)

20 mountain climbers (with 1-2-3-1, 1-2-3-2, 1-2-3-3, 1-2-3-4 . . . count)

Tuesday

Warm up on the elliptical machine with increased resistance level (five minutes)

15 weighted deadlifts at 45 lb. (your choice what type [e.g., sumo])

Isolation hold on deadlift (about 10–15 seconds)

Repeat cycle while decreasing weight by 10 pounds, until five sets are completed

In between the last few sets, perform 10 burpees, mountain climbers, and jumping jacks (e.g., after 15 repetitions of deadlifts, do 10 burpees), then after the next set of deadlifts, finish with 10 mountain climbers (count 1-2-3-1, 1-2-3-2, etc.), and final set of deadlifts, complete 25 jumping jacks

Wednesday

Walk the track or go to the park (one hour)

Ab work (five 30-second plank holds; bicycle crunches 45 seconds *times* five)

Thursday

Tire flips (choose your size that pushes you, but allows safe lifts)

Jump rope, light jogging around the track, or brisk walking (choose best option for you)

Alternate tire flips with jumping rope or your choice of above cardiovascular work

Friday

Workout routine from Monday or Tuesday (follow exactly)

If you choose to do a completely different workout, here is another sample option:

15 jump lunges on each leg (with or without ankle weights) (2.5 lb. or more)

15 weighted overhead press with dumbbells (choose a challenging weight, but not too heavy that you cannot complete a quality full overhead press—remember, you will complete this exercise at least three to four more times within your session)

25 crunches with extended legs and touching toes (with or without ankle weights at 2.5 lb. or more)

Running in place—sprint as fast as you can for at least 45 seconds *or* run as fast as you can and touch the imaginary line at least 15 yards (sprint drills). Sprints can be performed in yards ranging up to 100 yards at your maximum speed or effort. Choose the distance best for you but go hard!

Complete each of these exercises for at least three to five rounds for a full session

HIIT Benefits

High-intensity interval training (HIIT) has many benefits for you to improve your health. Your body has the opportunity to positively respond to the intense workouts designed for your HIIT workout plan. It is important to know that your overall goal is to help improve your current state of health and maintain a good health and fitness level throughout the year—every year for life! HIIT has been studied by researchers to show its benefits to your overall health and conditioning. Some of them will be summarized here, but there is much more to the benefits of HIIT.

Increase in VO2 max. The body requires oxygen for performance in exercise training. Specifically, HIIT can improve the body's ability to improve oxygen consumption. The muscles of the body require oxygen and nutrients during exercise to support workouts. As oxygen consumption increases and improves, the muscles can use oxygen and improve ability to perform intense movements. Muscle strength and endurance are important for HIIT performance, maintenance, and sustainability over time. When exercising according to the HIIT program, remember three words: volume, oxygen, and maximum. These words describe VO2 max which is your body's maximum rate of oxygen consumption during exercise (this can be measured).

Improve cellular mitochondria activity. The mitochondrion is the powerhouse of the cell within the body. It is responsible for the body's energy production. The body's overall health begins at the cellular level. The cells support and form all other parts of the body—the tissues, organs, and organ systems. HIIT supports this cellular energy powerhouse and improves its function. Think about it, good cellular energy support from your HIIT program will provide overall good fitness performance and health. Healthy cells, tissues, organs, and organ systems means a healthier and improved YOU!

Help fat loss and muscle gain. Remember, when you perform HIIT, you are taking your health and fitness to another level. You are doing more work—harder, more intense workouts in a shorter period of time. This intensity allows your body to burn fat calories from food, and that subcutaneous fat underneath the skin that you can grab, and the bad visceral fat that surrounds the organs inside of your body. Your body produces hormones such as catecholamines, cortisol, and growth hormone which all respond positively to the HIIT style, assisting your body in the increase in fat-burning hormonal activity and the reduction in negative stress response. That unhealthy fat must go, and your body is intelligent enough to produce the necessary chemical reactions to support that healthy fat loss process! As you take advantage of weight training and intense circuits in your HIIT workout plan, your body will increase in both muscle growth and reduction in unwanted, unhealthy fat. Yay!

Increase in metabolic rate. Your body is naturally a fat-burning machine. It has the ability to shed unhealthy fat, along with so many other processes that support overall health. Eating healthy and combining high-intensity exercises like

HIIT will help the body's natural ability to burn fat. Researcher have supported HIIT as a healthy way to reduce body fat when performed regularly each week and intense sessions of twenty minutes or more. So get your HIIT workout on and maximize your healthy fat loss!

Improvement in health conditions. Some of the leading causes of death and disability in the US and other countries includes diabetes and heart disease-related illness (i.e., high blood pressure, high cholesterol, high triglycerides, etc.). HIIT programs performed successfully over a period of time can support the body to improve these conditions naturally. Type 2 diabetes has been supported by health professionals to be preventable. HIIT can aid the body in improving blood sugar levels. It is also helpful in improving the body's resistance to insulin. People who have been classified as being overweight and obese can experience the benefits of decreased heart rate and blood pressure to healthy readings when continuing HIIT as lifestyle implementation programming. Get busy improving your overall health conditions and say bye-bye to preventable heart-disease risk factors and the conditions that increase its development—come on, you can do it!

Chapter 5

Nutrition Basics for You!

Six classes of nutrition include carbohydrates, lipids, proteins, vitamins, minerals, and water. These biochemical molecules or nutrients are necessary to sustain life and the biochemistry of the human body. Your body naturally contains these chemical substances required to sustain life. Some substances will be obtained from food sources to support the body's growth and development. Understanding the biochemical basics of your body's anatomy (the parts and how they are made—it's structure) and physiology (how these parts work—it's function) helps you better understand how the nutrients found in food support the body. Your body is made up of atoms which form molecules, which form cells that create tissues, that form the organs which make up your organ systems, that compose your complete organism—you!

Food provides energy in the form of calories. Energy from food is processed, stored, and used by your body's liver, adipose (fat) tissue, and muscle cells. When you consume food, you need to understand that you are eating food that can be digested or broken down into the nutrients they provide and the amount of those nutrients. Then, you must understand that your body will absorb a percentage (allow those nutrients to be carried into the bloodstream and be used to support your physical body requirements) dependent upon your current level of health. Different kinds of food provide different calorie amounts and contain substances that can help your body build lean muscle and burn unwanted unhealthy fat.

It is necessary to eat a variety of food that support your health and HIIT fitness goals. Dependent upon your nutrition practice (whether you are vegan, vegetarian, or neither of these and you consume meat or other substances provided by animal sources) will determine the food you consume, and the energy needs you meet. Vegan nutritional style and practice will have variation to the nutrients received by the body from sources other than animal sources (this could include meat from animals, eggs, dairy, and any other animal-derived products). Food sources that may be included in both vegan and vegetarian diets would include, but not limited to, tofu (substitute for animal meat made from soy to obtain protein), fruits and vegetables, various types of milk (e.g., almond, soy, rice, etc.), soy, legumes, beans, seeds, grains, nuts, and the list goes on. On the other hand, vegetarianism also has variations in nutritional style and practice. Some vegetarians consume some nutrients from animal sources such as dairy and eggs (i.e., ovo-vegetarian [eggs] and lacto-vegetarian [lactose from milk, dairy products]). The important fact is to combine food to obtain the necessary amounts of protein, carbohydrates, and healthy fats, along with vitamins and minerals to sustain a healthy nutrition plan necessary for good health.

Different lifestyles offer different styles of overall nutrition. These different styles will determine how meals are planned. The specific type of food, the amount consumed, and how food is prepared and the source from which it comes are all considerations in meal planning. Then, on top of that, consider the nutritional support necessary for an exercise regimen. Again, dependent upon a specific nutrition practice, the energy needs will vary, and meal plans can take on different styles. Importantly, ensure that your nutrition is supportive of your physical activity and specific HIIT fitness goals.

An example of a day's nutritional regimen (nonvegetarian or animal-derived source consumption) for a female athlete that supports the HIIT workout might mimic a nutrition style such as this:

Breakfast, Lunch, Dinner and Snack

8:00 AM–4:00 PM—intermittent fasting (IF)—*discussed in the next chapter*

4:00 PM—grilled salmon (3–4 oz.)

 ½ cup asparagus

 1 cup brown rice

 8 oz. cup of pure water

6:00 PM—grilled chicken salad (large)—mixed with almonds (or other nuts) and fruits

 8 oz. cup of pure water

8:00 PM—lean turkey breast (3–4 oz.)

 1 ½ cup broccoli

 1 small sweet potato

 8 oz. cup of pure water

10 PM—1 medium turkey burger patty

 1 ½ cup cabbage

 1 ½ cup green beans and potatoes

 8 oz. cup of pure water

Snack options may include brown rice cakes, fruit cup (natural fruit slices, not fruit in syrup), nuts (raw and unsalted rather than those with added sugar or sweeteners), no recommendation of high-sugar *sweet treats* such as cakes, cookies, pies, etc. During this time, the focus should be on developing the nutrition discipline for food (including beverages) not high in simple carbohydrates (i.e., sugar, syrup, etc.). The goal is not to focus on what you cannot do, rather what you can do. There are sweet treats designed for special nutrition that support healthy carbohydrate intake. Some of these may include cookies or other sweets with a high protein content and low net carbohydrate (total carbohydrate minus dietary fiber and low in sugar). At times, there will be an opportunity within the day that will allow carbohydrates—when the full day of eating has been low in carbohydrates to the point that a sweet treat snack will keep you within limits.

Gym time can be scheduled during the intermittent-fasting period or during the day at the preferred time of convenience. The HIIT workout should be focused on weight training with a mixture of cardiovascular-type exercises with low rest periods. For instance, a set of push-ups followed by a set of squats would be supportive of exercises that engage multiple muscle groups. Running in place for thirty seconds followed by abdominal work would allow the body to increase the heart rate with different exercises. The important thing is to keep moving while working different muscle groups that strengthen and movements that support fat burning. All exercise and other physical activities throughout the day should take into consideration the importance of maintaining a caloric deficit (calories consumed is less than calories burned) and should exceed the total amount of calories consumed. The idea is to burn more overall calories through exercise than is consumed nutritionally. For example, if your total calories equal 2,500, then you will want to make sure that your physical activity burns at least that much energy or more. Remember, the focus is on improvement in consuming quality calories from healthy food choices. Eat more quality food and perform high-intensity quality exercises. Give it your best in the kitchen and in your exercise sessions.

Focus Food Examples to Support HIIT

There are foods that can support your training goals. It is important to enjoy the food that you consume while still reaching your goals to include fat burning. You are likely aware of the extensive food list of fat-burning, high-fiber, muscle-building food available on the Internet. However, the most important fact is to find food that you love and new food that you can try to stimulate your natural body system processes that will help you get good results and fast! You may want to focus on food that assist your body's ability to burn fat because they contain substances that aid in this important metabolic process. *Some* of these foods (including beverage) may include, but are not limited to:

avocado	berries	chickpeas	egg (whites)	grapefruit
apples	banana	chicken	kale	lemon
almonds	broccoli	oatmeal	spinach	wild salmon
peppers	olive oil	lime	orange	asparagus
cucumber	pumpkin	coconut oil	brown rice	walnuts
turkey	sweet potato	tuna	green tea	onion

Water is absolutely the most important beverage to support all body processes.

Dietary Supplementation

Dietary supplementation is an important subject to familiarize yourself with when completing a HIIT program. Dietary supplementation is exactly what it reads, "dietary supplementation." It is designed to supplement, or complement, your daily nutrition plan. It is not to be used as a replacement for eating healthy food that support your training. You must allow the process of self-discipline to be an active part of your lifestyle—both for nutrition and exercise. Too many times, people tend to use dietary supplements to take over the lifestyle practice of eating a variety of food packed with vitamins and minerals and other substances naturally found in the body, plants, and animals.

The purpose of eating various types of food is because the human body naturally contains substances that support the body system processes that you require to assist you in achieving your personal fitness goals. Nothing compares to teaching your body to respond to the appropriate nutrition. It is key to understand that food, particularly dietary supplements, contain chemicals that will cause a chemical reaction to occur in the human body. The specific amount of a particular substance, the length of time you consume a particular substance, and your current body's state and level of health will determine your individual results. You cannot compare what your body does to that of someone else. There are many factors that contribute to your individual results when using a particular dietary supplement.

Your body is quite intelligent and knows what to do and how to adjust to getting in shape. It requires your support of getting fresh air, natural sunlight, pure clean water, physical activity, proper nutrition, and rest. Most importantly, it requires your patience in allowing it to respond naturally to its environment (mentally, physically, and spiritually). You are responsible for taking control of your life and doing what is necessary to provide the right atmosphere for your health. No one else can do this for you!

Yes, it is understood that there will be times when these important things get neglected with life and its daily routines. Nevertheless, dietary supplementation is only beneficial when offering support to your healthy lifestyle practices. Depending upon dietary supplementation to replace good habits of healthy nutrition practice could lead you to the disappointment of not achieving good results. Only lifestyle practices will support long-term sustainability. You want to continue to look and feel good after you get your results. Realistically, you know that what you don't continue can backfire on you (i.e., getting in great shape and then getting right back out of shape in just a few months because you didn't take the time to learn to change your lifestyle and develop healthy habits to maintain for life).

Dietary supplementation for HIIT should only come after you have become familiar with your daily training routines. You should learn to focus your attention on getting in the habit of working out regularly. Your attention should also be on developing consistency in saying your positive affirmations before and during the workouts each day. You can say them throughout the day because your mind needs to consistently know that you are determined to feel good about what you are doing to continue long term. Remember, HIIT is another level of fitness.

There are some dietary supplements that you can have as a supportive part of your HIIT protocol. These nutrients are naturally found in the human body. They can be found in plant food and meat (as well as alternatives to meat for those who are practicing vegetarianism or veganism). It is important to ensure that you consume a variety of food that contain these substances and know the amounts that you consume to know how much will be supportive for your dietary needs. These substances will be briefly covered in the "Questions of Consideration" chapter of this book.

Keeping Nutritional Balance

Now that you are aware of the important foods and nutrients provided to support human growth and development, you must consider the importance of balance. Nothing is ever perfect, especially in the learning process. There are new applications available for you to access to assist you with your fitness and nutritional tracking. There's so much talk about staying on track and not falling off your daily regimen. However, what happens if you do? What happens when you have a *cheat meal* or consume a considered *unhealthy sweet treat* or snack? You regroup! Don't beat yourself up.

First, congratulate yourself for growing enough to recognize a behavioral change that you would have neglected to notice in the past. Second, this is when you have to take a closer look at your *macros*, the nutritional protocol for the consumption of protein, carbohydrate, and fat for your recommended daily intake of calories per day. For instance, based upon a 2,000-calorie diet, you would calculate the calories you've consumed from your unhealthy sweet treat or cheat meal. Then, subtract those calories individually from the total amount per day that you must consume to stay within your total macronutrients. For example, if your goal is to temporarily restrict carbohydrates to 50 grams, then you will take that into consideration from the recommended total 2,000 calories per day. So as you continue your meals for the remainder of the day, consume food that allows you to stay within the amount of macronutrients you need to stay on track. No matter the food or beverage, you can maintain balance and still benefit. For example, if you ate a sweet bun with a total of 350 calories, 19 grams of fat, 42 grams of carbohydrates, and 4 grams of protein, you will have a remainder of 1,650 calories to fulfill your total calories of 2000 calories for the day. To do this successfully, you will likely consume mostly lean meats, vegetables, and healthy fats for the day. Remember, based upon a 2,000-calorie diet for the you're your recommended daily total fat should not exceed 65 grams to include 25 grams of saturated fat, and protein needs based upon pound per your bodyweight. Because you may be in carbohydrate restriction of 50 grams (according to this example) instead of the 300 grams as recommended daily, you will want to save your complex carbohydrates like brown rice, quinoa, sweet potato, or oatmeal for the next day. Instead, you can eat those vegetables like broccoli, asparagus, or other choice with less carbohydrate grams since you only have eight grams left before exceeding your target goal of 50 grams.

Third, take advantage of daily logging of your food, HIIT exercises, and other daily activities to guide you. Whatever your remaining meal plan, you will make sure the rest of your food (including beverage) is monitored closely. This is when calorie counting, nutritional tracking, and a fitness tracker (via a downloadable app) may be beneficial to assist you with knowing your daily intake versus your caloric output (how much physical activity helped you burn calories). Overall, maintaining a caloric deficit by consuming less calories (of course, while still maintaining a healthy caloric intake per day (e.g., 1800–2500 calories) than those you burn through your physical activity.

CHAPTER 6

Health Behaviors

Health behaviors are those activities and practices that you view as the actions taken to improve, maintain, and sustain overall health or prevent optimal health. There are various types of health behaviors dependent upon the field of study. They can be considered and accepted—both individually and societally—as good (supportive) or bad (hindrance) in their influence on health outcomes for better quality of life. Your personal choices during this HIIT challenge will provide encouragement and have the potential to offer the motivation necessary to impact overall results. This chapter is to encourage you to consider your personal beliefs about *your* current health behaviors—those things that you choose to do or not do to assist your mental, physical, and spiritual health and how it relates to your HIIT performance and ability to sustain this activity for better health.

As written in previous chapters, HIIT is the focus and goal.

This is a type of physical activity, which is considered and accepted as a healthy behavior. Other terms used in association with health behaviors are adverse health behaviors and risk behaviors. Physical inactivity is among the many terms referred to as an adverse health behavior. Research scientists have studied various types of health behaviors and the relationship and role they play in healthy outcomes. Adding HIIT to your daily lifestyle practices will allow you to participate and support your overall health-improvement goals. It is important to know that exercise is supported or hindered by specific lifestyle choices as will be discussed in this chapter. Key points for HIIT have been discussed in chapter 4 and other important information will be addressed later in this book.

Appropriate diet is important in supporting your HIIT and overall health goals. Your choice of meal preparation, routine, and food choices influence how you feel and how well you will be able to perform your new HIIT routine. Food provides you with energy to sustain the HIIT activity and improvement or prevention in current health status. Your personal beliefs and food choices must be considered as you accept this journey and how you benefit now and in the long run. The key points of healthy nutrition to support HIIT have been included in chapter 5, and other important information will be addressed later in this book.

Sufficient sleep is necessary to enjoy a positive experience during your HIIT performance and maintenance journey. Sleep is a healthy habit and behavior that allows the body to recover from full daily activities and HIIT exercises. Your body needs to benefit from significant amounts of rest each day. The importance of getting frequent sleep has been studied by researchers and how beneficial it can be for your health. Choose to prioritize sleep during your HIIT challenge and in your daily lifestyle practices.

Enjoy natural sunlight and fresh clean air during your HIIT experience. You can take advantage of performing your HIIT exercises outdoors. You can walk, jog, run, swim, play one of your favorite sports games, or whatever you choose. You have many options. Whether you choose to train in your backyard or your local park, there are many benefits to allowing your body to receive natural sunlight. Your body is designed to react to the natural sunlight. Did you know that your body produces vitamin D when exposed to the sun? That's just one benefit to your body's natural chemical reaction to the sun. You can enjoy the fresh, clean air by focusing on positive meditation during your exercises—whether it's for your warm-up or cool down or your rest periods between circuits. Take time to experience the great outdoors and enjoy the beauty that has been provided to you.

Hydrate your body with plenty of clean, purified water. Over 50 percent of your body is made of water. It is designed specifically to have water to maintain its health and well-being. All of your body's chemical reactions and processes require water. As you engage in your HIIT experience, make sure you remember to stay hydrated. Your body will perform at its best with sufficient water intake each day. Although many beverages include water as an ingredient or main component, do not consider other beverages as your calculation for appropriate water intake. For example, drinking tea or other drinks containing water is not the same as consuming water to be counted as those "eight glasses of water" each day. Remember, your activities may require more depending on many factors (i.e., how much water you lose throughout the day). No other beverage can take the place of water, so make sure you get water—plain, clean water, and plenty of it!

Now there are some health behaviors that may make it difficult for you to perform your best HIIT exercises. These may include those adverse health behaviors referred to earlier in this chapter. Research scientists have long studied the effects on health and these behaviors. They also must be considered in relation to how you will perform your HIIT exercises.

Two of them that you're likely familiar with would include, but are not limited to, smoking (secondhand or direct) and heavy or excess alcohol consumption. Smoking can influence a negative experience because you inhale carbon monoxide which travels through the blood to the vital organs of your body like the lungs. This can make it extremely difficult when considering how oxygen travels to the body to assist in overall body performance and especially hard, vigorous, high-level intense training like HIIT. In another example of consideration, it is recommended that you do not consume sugar or alcohol (or more specifically, engage in heavy drinking) for best results in most exercise and health and wellness programs. Excess alcohol consumption can affect your results for obtaining a lean body mass quickly and how you sustain your program over a period of time.

You want to use your body's energy to gain your best results, and faster. HIIT is expected to aid the body in burning a significant amount of body fat in a short period of time. Your daily habits and health behaviors will influence how you get the results you've been looking for and the time it takes to get there. Overall, HIIT must be considered based upon one successful session at a time, over a longer period of time. Your support for one individual session can be made easier or more difficult depending on your additional activities and health behaviors— just think about it for sixty seconds!

Health Behaviors: Positive Affirmations

I AM in control of my health behaviors.

I AM focused on the health behaviors that I desire rather than those I do not.

I AM happy to choose health behaviors that support good health.

I HONOR my body with healthy behaviors that improve my health.

My body was designed for me and deserves to be treated with love.

I have a happy, healthy body full of goodness and healthy behaviors daily.

I enjoy practicing healthy behaviors and my body responds positively to it.

I AM successful with healthy behaviors that benefit HIIT.

CHAPTER 7

Questions of Consideration

Metabolism and Your Body

Q: What is metabolism and how does it affect your body?

A: Metabolism is the sum of processes that occur in your body. Your body must build up and break down substances. Anabolism is the metabolic process that takes small molecules and uses them to form new larger molecules. Catabolism is the metabolic process that takes larger complex molecules and creates smaller molecules.

Glycogen-Store Depletion

Q: How long does it take to completely deplete your glycogen stores?

A: Glycogen is a form of energy. It is a polysaccharide (many glucose sugar molecules), which means that it consists of long chains of glucose (sugar molecule, energy to fuel your body). These chains are broken down to individual glucose molecules. Your body will require an average of one to two days to undergo this process. Once your body depletes its glycogen stores through normal physical activity and from exercise, you will begin to kick into that physiological level within your body that will assist your body in burning more fat for energy. Your body will get this energy from food that contain carbohydrate nutrients (sugars, starches, fibers).

Intermittent Fasting

Q: What is intermittent fasting (IF) and how can it be used to support training?

A: Intermittent fasting is a practice in which you follow an eating schedule, or time for the allowance of meals (eating window period) and a period that you do not consume food (fasting window period). During sleep, your body is in a fasted state. After waking, you enter intermittent fasting when you do not consume calories from food or beverage for several hours. There are different variations for the scheduled meals and time of fasting caloric restriction. For example, you may choose to restrict calories for a full eight hours after awaking from a full night's sleep. This will be translated to having sixteen hours of caloric restriction. During this time, you may complete your regularly scheduled training (of course, with caution because different effects occur based on individuality). Depending upon the time you wake up, you may choose to have your first meal of the day eight hours later. For instance, if you wake up at 6:00 AM, then you will consume your first meal around 2:00 PM. For your lunch break, you may choose to use that time to exercise. Then, that afternoon you will have your first meal of the day, followed by several meals throughout the day every few hours or so until about 10:00 PM. There are other examples that may involve less time for calorie restriction. You must choose the best option for you but having an eight-hour window for consuming calories is a great way to start. Remember, it is a practice so it will take some time to get adjusted—mentally and physically.

Intermittent fasting has been used to support training through the concept that as your body experiences low levels of insulin, it will be forced to use stored energy as a fuel source. This translates into your body burning unwanted, unhealthy fat for energy to fuel your activities—exercise or any other physical activities.

Exercises That Build Muscle and Burn Fat

Q: What examples of exercises build muscle and burn fat at the same time? What example of exercises are good for burning more calories?

A: Running (sprints), jogging, jumping rope, tire flipping (utilization of different sizes—large to small using good distance, e.g., 20 yards back and forth), weighted power deadlifts, full-body squats with overhead press with weights, burpees, row machine with focused speed, thirty- to sixty-second treadmill sprints with recovery walk (jogging on and off when unable to sprint and finishing with walking to keep movement of calorie expenditure—energy used by the body during your exercise activity).

Speed and Exercise Practices

Q: How can speed be increased and what exercise practices can be implemented?

A: Speed will come as you build your strength and endurance. The more you spend time with consistency in your cardiovascular work, the more you will increase your muscular strength and endurance. As you increase your weight training to improve stronger glutes, quadriceps, hamstrings, and calves, your overall leg power will follow. When you perform weighted upper-body work (chest, shoulders, biceps, triceps, back, and overall core muscles), you provide the powerful arm movement necessary to power speed. As you perform overall core muscles, which includes all areas of the abdomen, lower back, and spine and practice running on the track with no restrictions to your speed (in comparison to the treadmill); your heart muscle conditioning and increased blood flow through your vessels will provide you with the support to endure longer workouts and increased exercise performance for improved structural posture and strength to supply powerful movements, faster speed, and greater distance runs.

Six Pack and Belly Fat

Q: What is the best way to get a six pack or lose unwanted belly fat?

A: You want to focus your training on reducing your overall body-fat percentage. You will focus your attention on exercises that utilize your full body and allow you to utilize different muscle groups at the same time. You will want to increase your cardiovascular exercise with weights (examples listed above). As your body begins to reduce overall body-fat percentage, you can then focus your attention on muscle definition of the abdominal area. Remember, abdominal exercises will increase muscular strength and endurance in that area of your body. Body-fat reduction will take place from your entire body—not your abdominal area for spot reduction (thinking that your abdominal exercises will reduce the fat around the midsection or remove belly fat). You must focus your mind on reducing body fat from your entire body as it will allow you to see the muscle layer underneath the fat around the abdominal area. The abdominal workouts will allow the muscle to be built underneath the fat. So as the fat is reduced, the six pack will become more visible.

Take note that timing varies dependent upon the types of exercises completed with the nutrition to support muscle-building and body-fat reduction percentage through fat-burning routines. So how much time (days, weeks, months, years, etc.) does it take for *you* to visibly see your six pack abs? The answer to this question, *How long* is it going to take *you* the time it takes you is the amount of time that you clock when you see the six pack. For example, let's say that you've been successfully completing your health and fitness, lifestyle routine for six months and you see your abdominal area take shape exactly how you want—your six pack is completely revealed. Congratulations! You know that it took you six months. It may be less or more time for someone else. Do not compare your results with other people because there are many factors involved.

EPOC

Q: What does EPOC stand for and how is it defined?

A: EPOC is an abbreviation for excess post-exercise oxygen consumption. EPOC means that the body requires oxygen to utilize energy necessary for the exercise performed. The more strenuous the exercise, the more oxygen required to perform the exercise. The energy used to perform the exercise causes calories to be burned from food consumed or in the case of fasting, from fat storage. When exercises are performed with very little rest prior to moving to the next exercise—and the exercises are strenuous, requiring much energy, the body's oxygen is taken to fuel the body for full performance. Therefore, the body is still burning calories much later, after the exercise is no longer being performed. For example, you run sprints for sixty seconds, immediately begin doing twelve push-ups, then perform twenty-five squats with overhead press using ten-pound dumbbells, complete twelve energy-powered burpees, and end moderately jogging in place for thirty seconds. After, you repeat this cycle four to five times to represent a complete workout. This may take you ten minutes or longer to perform. Completing an exercise routine such as this for four or more days during the week would be an example of the EPOC effect on the body and its use of oxygen for performance.

Muscle Building and Fat Burning

Q: What role does building muscle play in burning body fat? How do you support healthy muscle growth?

A: Building muscle is important because the more muscle your body has the more body fat it will burn. Muscle weighs more than fat. It is denser in comparison to body fat. Adding more quality muscle to your body allows your body to burn more fat, even when you're not exercising. As you build your muscle over your entire body, you will increase your body's ability to perform at a higher level. You will be stronger, allowing you to lift, push, and pull more weight. Your body will be able to endure longer when performing exercises or daily activities. Physically, you will be able to see the muscle definition. As your muscle definition increases, the skin over the muscle will adjust and tightly hug the muscle underneath the skin. The body fat between the skin and muscle will decrease, allowing you to visibly see the muscle. This is where that pursuit for a leaner look and lower body-fat percentage become important to sports athletes and enthusiasts, as well as physique competitors.

Building the muscle must be supported by having a high-protein nutrition regimen. It is necessary to consume a protein amount that is enough to maintain current muscle and increase new muscle development. Whether you choose dietary supplementation, use a plant-based or animal protein, or other from natural food sources, you must consume healthy portions from lean sources to support such growth and repair. You must focus on consuming complex carbohydrates to support protein synthesis and fruits and vegetables high in fiber to support body-fat reduction and the overall process of elimination that help the body rid itself of unhealthy fat. Yes, you must eat!

As you build the muscle, the focus must be on increasing muscular strength, size, and endurance. It's important to focus your attention on compound movements that involve multiple muscle groups, particularly those large muscles of the body—which increase your body's efficiency at burning more calories and fat (increased metabolism). Exercises must include weight (bodyweight or other sources such as weighted bars, dumbbells, etc.) and repetitions and sets that will support these goals. For instance, you may want to increase a heavier weight and perform less repetitions and more sets, rather than use lighter weight and more repetitions with the same sets. Using a heavier weight that still allows you to safely perform the exercise will push your body harder and require it to do more work (or energy) to carry out the exercise. This will result in more oxygen usage and more energy required, and you will burn more calories as a result. Your workouts may be shorter in time, but the quality of work performed will make up the difference. Yes, you must put in the work—hard quality work to transform your physical body!

The exercises must be supported with the proper rest for repair of damaged muscle during the growth process. When you spend quality time building the muscle, the muscle fibers tear and must be developed in growth to come back bigger and stronger. This will require energy from your body, and you will be tired. So make sure you make time for plenty of rest. Yes, you must sleep!

Ketosis

Q: What is ketosis? How much sugar should you consume when on a ketogenic diet or to maintain a state of ketosis?

A: Ketosis is a metabolic process which is characterized by a state of low glucose availability in the body. As a response to low levels of glucose, the body's liver will react by producing substances known as ketone bodies which will be present in the blood and urine. When you do not consume carbohydrates from food, your body will not get the glucose as an energy source. There will also be a physiological response of low levels of insulin. Insulin is a hormone or chemical messenger that tells your body that there is too much glucose in the blood and will be released by your body's pancreas. Some physical activities such as HIIT that require your body to operate at a high physical intensity level, when you practice fasting (intentionally or unintentionally) or during long periods of sleep or rest, your body will find another way to maintain its energy to fuel your physical activities (both internally and externally)—using substances known as amino acids from protein and fatty acids from fat.

Carbohydrates such as sugar (natural sources such as those from plants, fruits, vegetables, cane sugar, honey, or added table sugar from certain food) are usually kept low on a ketogenic-friendly diet. Many foods like vegetables and fruits contain a natural sugar content while other food may add sugar to enhance taste. The amount of carbohydrates from these foods are monitored to limit the elevation of glucose so other sources can provide energy. It has been recommended by some professionals to select food with zero grams of total sugars or very little (it is important to note that some fat-burning healthy food such as broccoli naturally contain even as low as two grams of total sugars), no added sugars, or a maximum of twenty grams of carbohydrates in total per day. This number will vary from one health professional to another. As with anything, there are many factors to consider. For example, some people consider net carbohydrate which is determined by the difference between fiber (a carbohydrate source) and total carbohydrates (sum of all forms to include starch, dietary fiber, and sugar provided on a nutrition label including ingredients). Food and beverage provide calories for energy in these forms in varying amounts and must be considered. For instance, the net carbohydrate of a food source may be ten grams because the total carbohydrate is fifteen grams, and there is a total of only five grams of dietary fiber.

Dietary Supplements: Protein, L-Carnitine, and CLA

Q: What dietary supplements should be considered to support the HIIT program?

A: Dietary supplements that are supportive of the HIIT program include, but are not limited to, protein, L-carnitine, and conjugated linoleic acid (CLA). There are many supplements that are marketed for training intensively; however, these three supplements are the only ones that will be recommended at this time.

Protein is important because it is necessary for the muscle-building portion of your training. There are plant-based protein supplements (e.g., peas, seeds, sprouts, pumpkin, etc.) and animal protein supplementation (e.g., whey isolate or concentrate). You should know that the difference between whey isolate and protein supplementation is primarily the amount of protein, lactose, and milk fat. Plant-based protein comes from plant sources.

Whichever you choose, it is important to supplement grams of protein per bodyweight. For example, an active sports male or female athlete who weighs 120 pounds and is focused HIIT on building muscle would likely consume 0.8 to 1.4 to 1.7 grams per pound of bodyweight per day. The standard recommendation for an inactive person is 0.8 grams per kilogram of bodyweight or 0.36 grams per pound. The calculation for this 120-pound person would be 120 pounds multiplied by 0.36 grams of protein, which would equal about 43 grams of protein per day. This is standard and needs will vary dependent upon the intensity of muscle building and extreme athleticism. Careful consideration should be taken to ensure a variety of protein-containing food of choice provide protein supportive for energy requirements. Recommendations are to get your complete protein (protein that contains all nine of the essential amino acids) from food as much as possible and supplement when necessary to meet your needs supportive to your weight training.

L-carnitine is a substance that is naturally produced in the human body. It is also found in animal products such as beef (of course, you can consume lean grass-fed beef if you are concerned with beef consumption as a meat eater), eggs, cod fish and other fish, seafood, chicken, dairy, some vegetables, and grains. The primary function of L-carnitine is that it metabolically moves fat from storage and transports it to the mitochondria (powerhouse of the cell for energy production) where it can be utilized as an energy source. In a nutshell, it converts fat to energy. Yay!

Conjugated linoleic acid (CLA) is an omega 6 fatty acid which assists your body in utilizing fat for fuel. It is naturally produced from the essential fatty acid known as linoleic acid found in the oils of plants to support muscle maintenance while burning body fat. CLA is naturally found in many food sources such as dairy products (milk, cheese), meat (beef, recommended grass-fed beef), and plant products like safflower oil.

As you engage in your daily exercise routines in an effort to efficiently reduce unwanted, unhealthy body fat, your body will need to continue to support the precious muscle tissue that you've worked so hard to develop, strengthen, and define (tone and build).

Apple Cider Vinegar

Q: Does apple cider vinegar help burn fat?

A: Apple cider vinegar (ACV) is a natural substance produced from fermented apples. It contains a substance known as acetic acid which has been studied for its association with the chemical reaction produced by the human body, the hormone insulin and its role in body fat, as well as other important benefits. As mentioned earlier in this book, chemical substances found in food (including beverage) can stimulate the body's natural body system processes, causing a chemical reaction. ACV's acetic acid has been studied by researchers to show its effects on the body's ability to burn fat and provide a sense of fullness and aid in the suppression of your appetite, as well as improvement in insulin sensitivity. There are articles that have been summarized from peer-reviewed journal articles to give you insight on this nutrition.

Most importantly, you must understand that you must consider many factors in your individual physical-appearance results.

There are many contributing factors that play a role in your body-fat percentage just from apple cider vinegar alone. Your HIIT exercise program, nutrition regimen, water consumption, rest, overall stress levels, etc., are just a few of the factors to be considered.

CHAPTER 8

HIIT and Healing

Healing is a subject which cannot be neglected in this book. Healing must be considered when discussing HIIT. There are questions to take into consideration when performing HIIT and healing—healing from an injury. What if you sustained an injury prior to performing your HIIT workout program? What do you do now? How do you exercise when you have limited mobility? This section will discuss some options for you.

If you have limited mobility due to a prior injury or health condition which does not allow you to engage in the highest level of intensity, what do you do? You must alter your HIIT workout program. There is no need to be discouraged because you can still workout. You just have to change the way you work out. For instance, if you have difficulty with your knee health, you can alter the way you perform your compound movements (exercises which involve the use of multiple muscle groups at the same time). You can still work your full body by changing position. You can perform exercises which allow you to use your upper body and lower body in a different way. For example, you can do hanging leg raises which keep you from applying pressure to your lower legs. By holding your body weight with your arms, you can use ankle weights to lift your legs. You will determine how you choose to lift your lower body in a way that does not cause you discomfort. Depending upon the discomfort, you may choose not to bend your leg at the knee or keep it lightly extended. There are different ways to move around this kind of limitation, and only you can determine which is best for you. This way, you are in control and performing a full-body workout without the pain or difficulty. You can then perform push-ups, pull-ups, crunches, and other exercises which allow you to work other muscle groups. You can still perform those exercises at a high level, moving quickly from one exercise to the next with little to no rest.

You can apply this approach to any type of injury. Depending on the location of the injury, you will determine which body parts to use to maximize your performance during healing time. For instance, if you have an upper-body injury, you can also perform isolation exercises to engage the glute muscles (gluteus maximus, medius, and minimus) and hamstrings. Lie on your back or your stomach and allow the large muscles in your body to work. There is no specific way to improvise.

Remember, just get creative. Your body will always let you know what feels right. Use weights and do low repetitions or high repetitions with no weights at all. Just burn calories through quality work. Use all of the muscles you can when performing your exercises. Your body will still burn fat and build muscle in the areas worked. Take advantage of time. Learn how to do new exercises and movements that you may have never done before. You may need to use a support object like a chair, bench, or partner to assist you in completing the movements successfully. When you're determined, nothing will stop you!

One of the most important things that you must do when injured or going through the healing process is your nutrition plan. When you are unable to work at a high intensity due to injury, make sure you are eating right. Yes, you know what eating right means. And you must be strict! Because you are working with limited mobility, you have to depend heavily on your nutrition to support your muscle-building and fat-burning workout routines. You may not be able to burn as many calories per session. It will likely take longer to build muscle, too. So you have to eat food that support your goals.

Rest cannot be overstated. Get plenty of rest. Listen to your body. If you are not your best, allow your body to rest as much as you need to recover. Your body is designed to heal when you are sleeping. Give your body the time necessary to get back where it needs to be. When you allow your body time to recover, you come back stronger because you are able to perform at your best. Do not try to get back to your workouts without proper healing time. This can cause more injury and lead to more time away from your program goals. It's better to take a longer time to rest than to go back too early with a body which has not fully recovered.

Make sure to include your mindful exercises by performing your healing positive affirmations. This is the time to connect your mind and physical body. Before beginning your workout, close your eyes and think about the body's natural healing abilities. Envision the body healing in that area. See the cells and tissues working together as they were designed. Speak words of healing and positivity about your specific area of need. See yourself completely healed and continue to affirm, "I AM healed!" "Every part of my body is performing just as it was designed." "The cells and tissues of my body are anatomically and physiologically perfect." As always, you can choose to affirm the positive healing words of your choice. Believe what you are saying. Feel it from within. Keep your mind focused on achieving your goals. You will be guided in the area of performance. You will know what exercises are best for you. You will know the exact path to take to reach your ultimate healing manifestation.

HIIT and Healing: Positive Affirmations

I AM healed!

I have the mindset of healing.

I AM motivated to perform HIIT successfully with all of my healed body parts.

I AM focused on my healing from all injuries.

I think positively about HIIT and healing.

I see a positive outcome daily for my HIIT and healing transformation.

I feel the healing power within me that guides me to perform HIIT and all activities.

I continue to live in the space of good health and healing.

I AM emotionally healed from physical dysfunction.

I AM mentally, physically, and spiritually healed.

I have good thoughts about my healing.

I AM confident in the power within me to continue to be successful at living healed.

My attention is consistently directed toward maintaining positive healing.

I AM more than capable to perform HIIT and keep a positive healing mindset.

I AM enjoying the benefits of HIIT and healing as an overcomer.

No one can keep me down because I AM powerful!

Nothing can stop me because I AM healing power!

CHAPTER 9

HIIT Conclusion

In conclusion, HIIT is a style of training that gives your body a new level of health and fitness workout that is designed to shed that unwanted, unhealthy body fat and build a stronger physical body that's ready to achieve greatness. There is a lot of information provided in the book without too much technicality—which is the goal for readers. This is an additional resource to all the books and other resources available that get in more detail specific to HIIT. Spend time studying this information to learn more about your body and the options available to you to get the results you've been looking for.

It's important to make sure this book will not be another resource of a failed attempt to get you the physical transformation of your dreams. You must use the information provided to take you to your next level of health and well-being. You must understand that all it takes is your dedication and consistent practice to get real results. You are the one who will take you there, not just this book. Know that this is a new beginning for you. All the attempts in the past that did not yield the success you desired do not matter today. Forget about them and start over now! Stay encouraged with the positive motivation and inspiration provided—it's all here for you. Keep your focus centered on you and what you know you can achieve. Take one day at a time and keep it moving forward. Give yourself and your body the time necessary to become better than ever before. Remember, it's a process and it might not be as easy as you thought or imagined. Nevertheless, don't give up on you. You're definitely worth it!

Chapter 10

Enjoy and Balance!

This HIIT is a serious workout adjustment and is quite rigorous. It is important that you see it as a way to improve your physical state of health and fitness. There is much to do to get through each workout. You will be required to take it slow and easy. You must respect it as a goal to achieve each workout every day and until you reach the desired results.

Enjoy yourself! Do not take yourself too seriously to the point that you position yourself to fail. Sometimes, it's so important that too much pressure can be applied to the situation, and the activities will not be sustainable. Make sure to have fun with the exercises. Allow the challenges to motivate you to push even harder. Laugh at yourself when it gets tough rather than get frustrated and quit. You're not alone! Most people performing HIIT know how challenging and grueling it can be to complete an entire session. That's a part of it all! Allow that sweating, heavy breathing, and toughness to be the confidence you need to know you're getting to the next level.

Balance yourself and the process. Every process must have the respect and appreciation of balance. You must know that this is one part of an entire process to get you where you are going in your next-level health and fitness journey. If you overdo it, you might become too overwhelmed. All is required is that you give it your all and do your best. Give it your 100 percent maximum effort. When you need to rest, rest! When you need a day of rest between exercise days, when it is a prescheduled workout day, just go for a long relaxing walk. When you eat something that you believe is not supportive of the training, quickly deal with it and just move on. Recognize that there will be challenges to the adjustment phase. That's why you must continue to understand that it's a practice and one part in the lifestyle of health and wellness within your fitness plan. Keep the balance by not being too restrictive or too hard on yourself when you "miss the mark" in an area. Respectfully, that comes with it. Success always requires balance, and there's no other way to introduce, continue, or maintain HIIT. Keep your balance and keep it moving forward!

CHAPTER 11

Bringing HI*IT* Altogether

In this chapter, you will be guided on the conclusion of this entire book's important points that will help you understand the overall significance of HIIT for your personal physical results. You will have your attention centered on the way you think, feel and believe, speak, as well as create an atmosphere of positive and good HIIT results to successfully transform your body for health and wellness. Now that you have covered the basics of this book's information, you will be positioned to consider how you feel right now about that information. This is a very important section of this book and will determine your benefits of successful action toward a sustainable lifestyle practice. According the intention of this work and aim for total achievement of results, there will be personalized considerations of thought specifically for you.

What are your thoughts at this very moment about you and your expectations for beginning your HIIT journey at this time in your life? From the guidance offered in the previous chapters of this book, you have been provided with the basic information and tools for the successful application of HIIT readiness. You have positive affirmations to think about to encourage you to challenge your focus about HIIT in the direction of your actions to come. Your thoughts about HIIT prior to reading this book have been positioned in your mind for consideration at this time. Now you are here at the end and should be aware of what you think you can do, what results you think you will have at the end of your HIIT training implementation, and who you will be in reference to your confidence to transform physically, mentally, and spiritually in comparison to who you were on those levels. Do you think you can do it? Do you think you will do it? Do you think you will be consistent until your personal results have been achieved? Do you think you will continue with its incorporation as part of your personal lifestyle practice? The goal is to have positively good thoughts right now about your HIIT journey and future maintenance. Good questions, a lot of questions are all necessary to determine what you feel—now that you have been introduced to your thoughtful consideration of this book's content thus far.

How do you feel about the high-intensity interval training idea for you? What are your feelings about what you are about to experience with HIIT? Do you feel excited, nervous, intimidated, encouraged, etc., to begin this journey? Your personal feelings matter. Yes, at the end of your reading experience, you're guided to discover how you feel about what you've been doing so far—your previous exercise experiences, present physical condition, and your abilities for successful HIIT readiness and sustainability over the next several days, weeks, months, and lifestyle. The information that has been offered to you in this book is for your benefit toward successful action. The purpose is to result in HIIT action over time that will produce a habit to produce physical transformation. Your previous feelings and how you feel now should be different concerning you and HIIT for you. The goal is to feel good, comfortable, and confident about the HIIT journey and future maintenance. Once again, good questions, a lot of questions are all necessary to determine what you believe you can benefit from HIIT right now.

Do you truly believe that you can benefit from HIIT right now? The information provided in this book should position you to consider what you believe to be possible for you concerning HIIT. You should know that what you believe about yourself, and HIIT makes the difference between the successful action of getting started, continuing, and maintaining your HIIT practice. The goal is that you believe you can do it against all odds and will be successful for a higher level of physical transformation. After consideration of these questions, your present belief is necessary for acting required for you to speak the positive affirmations with confidence along your HIIT journey and its sustainability.

Are you speaking the positive affirmations with confidence? These are words of encouragement and power. You should be thinking about yourself and your HIIT experience through the action of speaking positively. You should be repeating them more and more until you feel comfortable speaking them. The words and the energy produced from them should begin changing your atmosphere. You should be more aware of the words you were speaking and those you're speaking right now. There should be a personal expectation of witnessing a physical difference. The goal is on positively speaking words about yourself, your HIIT journey, and successful maintenance. There are a lot of positive affirmations provided to speak directly about you, and they're all necessary to create an improved, mindful attitude for an atmosphere of change in the right direction for personal physical environmental benefits.

What atmosphere have you created in your mind and physical environment to prepare you for positively benefiting from HIIT? Now that you have received information in this book, what steps will you take now to create a positive atmosphere? The information within has already offered you the opportunity to think differently. Your mind has been focused on the words you will speak about you and HIIT. The positive affirmations will be repeated in your thoughts and spoken from your mouth. This will create an atmosphere of actions that should motivate and inspire you to create physical movement toward your HIIT experience. Now you should be surrounded by people who are supportive of your determination to improve your overall health and fitness or who are actively working toward their health and wellness improvement; exercise equipment supportive of your HIIT workouts, listening and watching positively uplifting messages; increased awareness of your HIIT exercises, workout routines, and practices that get your heart rate increasing, blood pumping through your body and transporting vital nutrients to your cells; and your growth and support necessary to visibly see physical transformation (muscle tone, energy production, decrease in body-fat percentage, etc.). The goal is to perform HIIT at home or the gym, be consistent, and keep getting better physically—stronger, leaner, and faster.

CHAPTER 12

Celebrate Your Success!

Now you are here and it's time to celebrate your success! You have reached the end of this book, and you must give yourself a pat on the back for completing it. Although you may be thinking that you have not done anything, yet you are well on your way. The first step has been completed for your new task. You have the information, and you are getting ready to put it into action right now.

Celebrate your first day of completing the mindful-practice exercises and each day thereafter. Remember, you will only take it one day at a time. You must make it your personal business to celebrate yourself along the journey to your successful completion of any part of this new training. If you are not new to HIIT, then you still must consider this moment differently because it is a new time for your training. You may be implementing a new routine for your HIIT workouts in comparison to the past. Your mindful-practice exercises may not have been a part of your training. Now, you are celebrating the focus that is being directed toward your exercises. You must take the time to feel good about what you are doing. There are other things you could be doing at this time in your life, but you are training your body to move faster, become stronger, and get leaner.

Celebrate the vision of successful completion of the new routine. It is extremely important to ensure that you envision yourself completing the workouts each day before you actually start. See yourself following through with each part of the program and crossing the finish line as a winner! Activate the thoughts and positive feelings associated with completing each repetition, set and eating the right way to support your growth. All is important, and nothing should be overlooked, underappreciated, or devalued about your success. Remember, you are successful. Now follow through with the actions to prove it to yourself. Congratulations! You're finished reading this book and now ready to get the results you've been waiting for!

PUBLICATIONS

Cole, LaKeisha J., Rohrer, James E., and Schulze, Frederick W. (2011). "Academic worry and frequent mental distress among online doctoral students." *ProQuest/ UMI Publishing.*

Rohrer, James E., Cole, LaKeisha J., and Schulze, Frederick W. (2012). "Cigarettes and self-rated health among online university students." *Journal of Immigrant and Minority Health, 14(3), 502-505.*

Other Books

From Failure to Success: Faith Changes the Outcome. 2019
Child, You Are a Sower: Plant Seeds of Goodness. 2020
Learning About Nutrition: Just for Kids. 2020
Learning Letters with Animals: Just for Kids. 2020
Numbers and Shapes: Just for Kids. 2020

Website

www.thefaithoutcome.com

YouTube

True Wellness Consulting, LLC

Dr. LaKeisha Cole